Musing and Muttering...

THROUGH CANCER

DAVID GAST

MUSING AND MUTTERING . . . THROUGH CANCER

Copyright © 2007 by David Gast

ISBN-10# 1-897373-18-X
ISBN-13# 978-1-897373-18-7

Printed by Word Alive Press
131 Cordite Road, Winnipeg, MB R3W 1S1
www.wordalivepress.ca

WORD ALIVE PRESS

*To all who are going through
difficult experiences,
especially those
on the cancer journey.*

*My desire is that
you will be encouraged,
and recognize
God's immense love for you.*

TABLE OF CONTENTS

ACKNOWLEDGEMENTS

A Special Thanks To . . .

The Canadian Cancer Society—for vigilant care of cancer patients and promotion of research to find a cure for this dreaded disease.

The Cancer Clinic, Soldiers Memorial Hospital in Orillia, Ontario—for highly professional and caring staff administering help to the helpless and hope to the hopeless.

My health care workers—doctors, nurses and others, for consistently giving me the best of care, always treating me as a real person.

Sharon—my wonderful wife, for being my principal care giver through the good times and the bad, lovingly encouraging me in this project, editing the script, and managing the many details related to its publication.

All my friends and family—for being a constant source of courage and joy through prayer, phone calls, cards and e-mails.

First Baptist Church in Orillia, Ontario—for caring for us in so many practical ways, and especially the choir for the delicious meals.

Dr. Gord Martyn—for being someone I could talk to when I needed special encouragement and counsel.

Jack Slade—my friend and 'designated driver' to many appointments, for not only providing transportation, but offering great companionship and encouragement.

The staff of Word Alive Press—for guiding me in the publishing of this my first book.

"I complained some. Not a lot, but more than enough! I also laughed some. God seemed to place outside my window things that could not be ignored. His graphic life lessons through birds and animals and wind and rain spoke to me of coping, and hoping, and rising above. You will discover these in the following pages as I mused and muttered along on my cancer journey."

PROLOGUE

WE ALL GET SICK with something or other from time to time. Just like me, I bet you're dealing with a negative physical issue or two right now. Funny how they call a diagnosis "positive" when it's bad, and "negative" when it's good. I never could figure that out.

One of my earliest recollections of being really sick was when our whole family got the mumps. You know how it happens. Kid one gets sick, then kids two and three, and then mom and dad. We were one miserable, puckering, mumpy bunch. Our inflated glands made us look like Sumo wrestlers from the neck up. It even hurt to laugh. Whoever came up with "mumps" for a name certainly had a sense of humour. To make things worse, my dad came up with the novel idea of each of us drawing our own depiction of what a real live mump might look like. We all just about died laughing!

Around that same time, I was being observed by my family doctor for another kind of lump in my neck—two of them. For three years they watched them develop only to find out that I had a malignant cancer. At age eleven I underwent major surgery followed by several months of cobalt bomb radiation. The "Baby Bomb" for kids was developed but had not yet arrived at the hospital, so I got a powerful dose from the Big Bomb. One day I remember being taken into a doctors' forum. Someone asked how much thyroxin I was taking. Wanting to impress these men of learning, I blurted out, "Two grams". Everyone burst into laughter. It was ".2 mgs"! That was 1955. I was eleven. Little did I know that fifty years later I would be given care and counsel by a dear friend and retired doctor, Dr. Gord Martyn, who had studied under my surgeon's tutelage and most likely had been in that very meeting.

The following winter I was allowed to play hockey. One of the other kids skated over to me and said, "What are you doing here? I thought you had cancer." Not until that moment did I realize that I had cancer. When I got home I asked my mother about it. She very sensitively explained the whole thing to me. Then it dawned on me. That was why The Canadian Cancer Society was so involved with my parents giving help with rides and financial assistance. That was why I had been going to the Cancer Clinic at Victoria Hospital in London for cobalt treatments. That was why Mom and Dad had told me that the whole church had organized an all night prayer meeting for me the night before my surgery. I began to realize how gracious God had been to me in sparing my life.

Ten years later I was given a clean bill of health. In that final check-up, they asked me what I was studying in college. I said I was studying music. "What's your major?" "Singing", was my nonchalant reply. "That's incredible", they said, "because we had to go in so close to your vocal chords with radiation and we didn't know if you would even be able to talk." That statement impacted me for the rest of my life, and I determined from then on to use my voice to the glory of God in whatever capacity He would lead me. I have just recently completed forty years of music ministry.

But my journey included a recent bout of lung cancer that was discovered in the Fall of 2004. Two surgeries and chemo therapy brought about significant changes in my life. At the time, I had no idea to what extent my life would be rearranged. But going down that path offered more "free time" than I can ever remember having. Time to ponder. To pray. To write. Time to observe God's creation. To assess life. To try and make sense of things that just didn't add up.

I complained some. Not a lot, but more than enough! I also laughed some. God seemed to place outside my window things that could not be ignored. His graphic life lessons through birds and animals and wind and rain spoke to me of coping, and hoping and rising above. You will discover these in the following pages as I mused and muttered along on my cancer journey.

This book is based on a collection of e-mails that I sent to "My Contacts" over the ensuing three years. Thanks to many of you for clicking on "Reply to Sender", encouraging me to publish them.

THE BATTLE

FACING CANCER IS LIKE facing an army. You have to put up your defenses, pull out whatever artillery is available and aggressively eliminate what would otherwise eliminate you. Only thing is, you can't see the culprit. It hides in our body tissues sometimes undetected. When the body fails to eliminate the enemy through its immune system, these tiny cells survive and grow by constant cell division. To beat the enemy, drastic measures often need to be taken, cutting them out or attacking these dividing cells through radiation or chemotherapy. The timing of the attack becomes crucial—the earlier the better.

Our first assault in the battle was the ultimate eradication of the obvious. Various tumours in my right lung were extracted in two surgeries, Oct. 19, 2004 and Jan. 4, 2005. After numerous scans, biopsies, x-rays and procedures, Dr. T., thoracic surgeon, was absolutely marvelous in his whole approach. He has given Sharon and me a high level of confidence and appreciation for the medical help available to us in Canada. But even after very successful surgery in which he removed the infected lower lobe of my right lung, and even though he said my lungs look very healthy (nice and pink mainly resulting from being a non-smoker), he made it clear that chemotherapy was an absolute necessity. It is what is not seen that can be of greatest danger.

The local Cancer Clinic will be one of the other key battalions in our army fighting this hideous disease. Yesterday, February 2nd, 2005, Dr. B., my oncologist, very kindly and sensitively outlined the details pertaining to ongoing treatment. He made it clear that there is great urgency here. The ammunition for battle against these pesky cells is a cocktail of chemicals called "Cisplatin" and "Vinorelbine Tartrate" that will be administered by intravenous injection. The dose will be very strong and will be administered weekly for 16 weeks. This was a surprise to me, but I appreciate the thoroughness. The first treatment in mid February will indicate a lot as to whether I can sustain this treatment and to what extent my immune system will be weakened. At the end of our consultation yesterday, Sharon and I both received a warm sincere hug from the attending nurse. It brought tears to my eyes to sense the care that obviously goes way beyond their call of duty. I may even look forward to treatments just for the hugs!

My ability and availability for work and ministry will be heavily curtailed during these next four to six months. I am to avoid any possibility of infection. Contact with a simple cold germ could develop quickly into pneumonia in my already weakened lung. My immune system may be reduced, because any fast dividing cells such as hair and the white and red blood cells are also attacked by the chemotherapy. They are like civilian casualties! The white blood cells determine our immune system, so if mine are heavily reduced, I may be advised to avoid crowds altogether.

The bottom line is that the ultimate battle is not medical, even though these procedures are of principle importance. The battle is the Lord's. I was reviewing the story of another battle in the Bible—II Chronicles, chapter 20. Jehoshaphat faces what appeared to be an impossible enemy. So God's people went to the Lord in prayer. The funny thing is that He ordered the music director and the choir to go to the front of the battle line and sing! I'm trying not to read too much into this! In verse 15 we read:

> This is what the LORD says to you: 'Do not be afraid or discouraged because of this vast army. For the battle is not yours, but God's'.

Then they headed out to fight, and found out that God had already beaten the enemy before they had to engage in bloody conflict. Then there was a great party!

Well, it is the same for me. I have never in my life had so many people praying for me. What a huge blessing and honour. E-mails and cards and phone calls from friends and family and connections bring heart-felt support and prayers. I am truly humbled. So whatever happens, I know that the Lord is in it. He will win this battle and bring about a result that glorifies Him. The battle is the Lord's. I am the Lord's—and victory is however He defines it. There will be a great party of thanksgiving, and we will all give thanks to the Lord for He is good.

In Philippians, which I quote by memory on my walks, a section impressed me this morning as being my thoughts exactly:

> *Yes, and I will continue to rejoice, for I know that **through your prayers** and the help given by the Spirit of Jesus Christ, what has happened to me will turn out for my deliverance. I eagerly expect and hope that I will in no way be ashamed, but will have sufficient courage so that* now *as always **Christ will be exalted in my body**, whether by life or by death. For to me, to live is Christ and to die is gain. If I am to go on living in the body, this will mean fruitful labour for me. Yet what shall I choose? I do not know! I am torn between the two: I desire to depart and be with Christ, which is better by far; but it is more necessary for you that I remain in the body. Convinced of this, I know that I will remain, and I will continue with all of you for your progress and joy in the faith, **so that through my being with you again your joy in Christ Jesus will overflow on account of me**.*
>
> ~Philippians 1:18b-26

So that's the journey as we are experiencing it at present.

WAITING AND HOPING

WAITING IS SUCH A CHALLENGE. Being still is not part of the agenda that I am used to. I don't know about you, but I naturally resist inactivity. Being involved and busy is a value that I have deliberately nurtured over the course of my life. You know what it is like, having an agenda that is seldom fully met and in which you have to choose priorities, always leaving trivial pursuits to fill the cracks of another day.

I have been in a waiting mode since mid February for treatment to continue, because the first chemo treatment really knocked me down. My strength is slowly returning, and the oncologist is holding off until early April before continuing. He is adjusting the chemicals hoping to find a mix that my system will tolerate.

I am learning to wait and be still these days— not an easy lesson for me! I have a lot to learn from Psalm 46:10 and the old familiar Psalm 37:7 which says:

"Be still, and know that I am God

"Be still before the LORD and wait patiently for him."

Could this mean that I actually come to understand God and His purposes in my life better when I am still and in a waiting mode?

When we served in Ecuador, we learned that the Spanish word *esperar* is the same word used for "to wait" as the word used for "to hope". In *Romans 8:24-26* the word wait is connected to hope. It says: *"For in this hope we were saved. But hope that is seen is no hope at all. Who hopes for what he already has? But if we hope for what we do not yet have, we wait for it patiently. In the same way, the Spirit helps us in our weakness."* This encourages me because in my waiting, I am also hoping that the Lord will bring me through, completely free of this hideous disease. I can't see the end result as yet, but I do "hope in the Lord", and thus I leave it up to Him.

So here I am. Waiting—learning the lesson of stillness and relative inactivity. It could drive me nuts were it not for the fact that I am really low on energy. It is so easy to sit down or lie down and sleep. My body tells me continually that there are limits to the energy pool. But I have discovered casual reading all over again, and that's a good thing as I face a stack of books that have been waiting a long time for me to crack open.

I lost 20 pounds. Yeah! But now the doctor is asking me to gain some weight! Me? Gain weight? This is a first. I'd almost rather not, since I'm finally down to what doctors in the past have said is an ideal weight for me.

It will be a few months before I can even hope to be back to work full time. In the meantime I try to keep contact with those who are carrying on leadership roles at the church. I miss being there all the time, but occasionally I show up for a rehearsal or a Sunday service as the Lord gives me strength.

Waiting and hoping in the Lord. For what? That remains to be seen.

MAYBE — JUST MAYBE!

TODAY, APRIL 13, I had my third chemo treatment. Maybe if I had tolerated the first one on Feb. 11 as well as I did last week's, I would have been up to number 10 of the 16 required. Maybe the first one was too much too soon. Or maybe my overall health and stamina is better now, having had almost two months to gain strength before going on.

Is "maybe" a word you tend to use as I do? There are days when I think it is a great word! Then there are other days! Maybe "maybe" leaves too many doors open in the doubting "what if" barn, especially the door of conjecture. Conjecture is an opinion based on incomplete information. Simply put, it is a guess.

Maybe I just like to try figuring things out, asking: What has happened here? Or what may have been if so and so hadn't happened? Maybe on the surface it is a gross waste of time. But I seem to have lots of time these days, so why not ponder the journey of life and get a broader perspective on where I am, where I've been and certainly on where I'm going?

For example, here I am, a non smoker with lung cancer, perhaps caused by radiation that I received for thyroid cancer in 1955. They had to use the big 'adult" cobalt bomb on me because the smaller baby bomb, though on order, had not yet arrived. Maybe if it had arrived, I would not be in this condition today. Or maybe, since it was paramount that I receive immediate treatment back then, just maybe I would not have made it at all had they waited. Only God knows.

One thing I do know is that back in the 60's when the doctors told me that they didn't think I would be able to talk because of the radiation near my vocal cords, I valued my gift in singing more deeply and dedicated my life to serve the Lord in music ministry. Maybe if cancer had never shown up, I would not have ended up in the ministry! Maybe I would never have met Sharon. Maybe I would have remained on the farm. Who knows? It's anyone's guess.

Certain things we may try to guess, but there are certain things we need to know. Here's one of them. With God there are no maybes. This is why He asks us to be decisive and let our yes be yes and our no be no. That forces us to enter into a trusting relationship with Him. He is committed to our best interests, bringing about in our lives what is good for us and what brings glory to His name. *Romans 8:28 (NLT)*, brings this truth into the foreground for me:

For we know that God causes everything to work together for the good of those who love God and are called according to his purpose for them.

Now, that really brings things into perspective. This is not a maybe, or a wild guess. This is something I know for sure, because it is a promise from God himself.

Maybe if I were to pursue a few more "maybe" scenarios, I would realize even more that only a loving God can make sense of it all. Maybe you too have a pocket full of maybes that leave you with many questions and cause unwanted doubts to pile up. Go ahead and think about them for awhile, and then let them lead you full circle back to a full trust in Jesus our Lord who is full of grace and truth—no guess work with Him. He knows the end from the beginning and has only your best interests in mind. Then maybe—just maybe—the next crisis in life will be seen from God's perspective.

DAYS COME AND DAYS GO

DAYS COME AND DAYS GO. Have you noticed recently how quickly a day evaporates? Morning propels us into familiar routines. There is always much to do and to accomplish. Each day unfolds event by event, task by task, but not always as we planned or expected.

I just came off two weeks of no chemo treatments due to a reduced immune system—often a side effect of chemotherapy. The white blood cell count which should be no less than 3, fell from 2.6 to 1.6 and then to 0.6. All the while my impatient inner clock was ticking. Even though my strength began to return, not having weekly treatments in my system, I was frustrated that it meant extending the overall treatment schedule into August or later, and watching the days incessantly come and go .

Yesterday, May 17th, I was sure that the numbers would still be down and I would not be permitted to go for another chemo treatment. But guess what! I got a call at 8:05 a.m. that it was a go. Those little white cells had bounced back to 2.9. So here I am back on stream with only 10 more treatments scheduled. I am responding well to the treatments with very little nausea. Loss of energy and stamina are constant realities, and I have been placed on full medical leave from the church. We are hoping it is not going to be for very long, but that is where I must be patient as the days come and the days go.

Just before Moses died and before the children of Israel crossed into the Promised Land, he gave a blessing to each of the 12 tribes. This is what he said to Asher:

> *Your strength will equal your days. The eternal God is your refuge and underneath are the everlasting arms.*
>
> ~Deuteronomy 33:25b, 27

As we face an uncertain future, and as tough days come and go, God will give the strength we need for each day. He will hold us in his strong arms. And that goes for you too!

As we live and breathe and move through each day, time is life, and life is time. Each is a gift from God, and we are stewards of them both. What I do with them says a lot about who I am and what my values are. At the end of the day—energy spent and emotions drained—one is left to ponder the significance of today in the scope of a life time. Just another day? A significant day? Or a lost day?

God views days from a much larger perspective than we do. He is patiently waiting for all of us to turn from our own ways and draw near to Him. Notice the words of 2 Peter 3:8-9:

> *But do not forget this one thing, dear friends: With the Lord a day is like a thousand years, and a thousand years are like a day. The Lord is not slow in keeping his promise, as some understand slowness. He is patient with you, not wanting anyone to perish, but everyone to come to repentance.*

As days come and days go, it is almost impossible to remember all the events of yesterday let alone a week or month ago. Only the highlights of today are fresh, yet soon to become fading memories of the tasks and duties that occupied our time and energy. The key thing that I am still trying to learn is to glean God's best for me each day by accepting His schedule and His events in His good time. May my prayer be that of David in Psalm 90:12 and 14:

> *Teach us to number our days aright, that we may gain a heart of wisdom. Satisfy us in the morning with your unfailing love, that we may sing for joy and be glad all our days.*

ANNOYANCE FROM HELL

THE OTHER DAY I was thinking about the Apostle Paul coping with his thorn in the flesh. Whatever malady that actually was, it was enough of an annoyance and inconvenience for him to ask God three times to take it away. I too have been there, done that, as you probably have as well. You can read about it in II Corinthians 12 beginning at verse 7. Its purpose was to keep him humble and the annoyance is described as a "messenger from Satan". I wonder how many annoyances in our lives are messengers from Satan, allowed by God to keep us humble.

Behind our house is a wooded area filled with beautiful, singing birds, many of which feast at our bird feeders. During these endless days at home coping with ongoing chemotherapy and wishing life was back to normal, my spirits are picked up every day as I sit and admire this piece of God's creation. The songs of the birds, so varied, so full of life and energy and so crystal clear, far excel any song I can sing. And as they stop by at the feeder, usually taking turns in groups according to species, I sit and admire them. I truly love them all—except one.

No, I am not meaning the black and blue grackles with attitude. Like big black bullies they barge in and demand their turn, temporarily scaring off the innocent little red and yellow finches. No, but there is one bird that is either directly sent from the pit of hell, or is brain damaged from pecking incessantly on the wrong things—like the eaves trough right outside our bedroom window. You guessed it. It's a woodpecker—to be specific, a downy woodpecker wearing a cute little red cap that reminds me of a flame from Hades. I call him Mr. Downer, because he is the biggest downer in my life. Even bigger than lung cancer. He is eating away at my patience and disturbing my sleep time! How dare Mr. Downer be so insensitive to someone on chemotherapy who is supposed to get his rest!

It would be one thing to hear a woodpecker peck away on a rotten tree for a reasonable duration, looking for his early morning snack of grubs and beetles. But it's something else to be rudely awakened at 4:30 a.m. with a blast of "Rat-a-tat-rat-a-tat-tat-tat-tat-tat" on the metal eaves trough, resembling nothing less than a machine gun. Once would be endurable. Time after time after time after time gets really annoying. Each time lasts for about three or four sets of ten taps. Then he stops for 15 minutes. Then he starts again, ad nauseum, continuing throughout the day. I should try some of my anti nausea pills for the ad nauseum part, and Mr.

Downer should be on Prozac. He is nothing short of a messenger from Satan.

This morning was the same routine. So after breakfast I decided to take action. I went out on the deck just below the eaves trough which extends along the back of the house. I sat in a chair reading a George MacDonald novel only to be interrupted by Mr. Downer down at the other end of the house. So I picked up a big stick and ran along the deck toward him, banging the eaves trough above my head. He quickly flew away. That should take care of the culprit, I mused.

No sooner had I gotten settled and half way down another page but there he was again, same routine but this time with more gusto. The next time I told him straight out, "Get lost. Be gone". The third time, I was sure he would never be back. Three times! Somewhat like the Apostle Paul, except I wasn't bothering God about it. I was going straight to the source. But this bird didn't get it. When I indicated clearly that he was to leave, I meant FOREVER!

After some time of no return, I decided to finish planting the garden. Immediately upon getting everything organized, I worked out front planting "impatience" plants. All of a sudden I was fully aware that Mr. Downer had returned to the back of the house doing his rat-a-tat. He thought I didn't notice, but I had work to do.

Lunch time had passed so I cleaned up and went back inside. "Rat-a-tat-rat-a-tat-tat-tat-tat-tat". So what am I to do, ignore him? Mr.

Downer needs boundaries. I strode out to the deck, looked him straight in the eye, and this time he looked back. Then he looked at the eaves trough. I banged the side of the house. He looked at me, and then again at the eaves trough. I banged even more loudly and shouted, "Get out of here you crazy bird" (or something like that!). He looked at me and then made three short taps and flew off. I may have been imagining it, but it seemed his head was turned toward me as if to say, "Gotcha again."

I sat down to write this little story, and three times I have been interrupted. Each time I went out to the deck, took my stick and aggressively walked towards the fiend. Each time (except the last one) he looked at me and nonchalantly flew off. The last time, two minutes ago, he did a hit and run. I heard him. I got up to scold him but he flew off before I could get there. When is he going to discover that trees are less wear and tear on the brain for us humans, and that eaves troughs don't store food?

O rats, there he is again. This time I'm going to ignore him and see if that works! Maybe God's humbling routine is working on me, be it ever so gradually.

THE WIND

IN MY LAST LETTER I complained about Mr. Downer, my woody woodpecker friend who insisted on pestering me endlessly, pecking on the eaves trough. A few hours after writing that letter, he took to moving from house to house, just stopping by my place when he knew for sure I was resting. Recently it appears that his campaign of neighbourhood annoyance has ceased.

It wasn't because I prayed against him. I felt it unwise to ask the Creator to turn against His own creation! I may have preyed *on* him a bit, teaching him that mankind is the dominant species of the universe and not to be trifled with. However, I am the one learning the lessons here. God appears to be teaching me how to become more tolerant and appreciative of these pressure points of life. And that's a good thing.

What really got my attention was Mother Downer eating from our bird feeder and feeding her young woody from the same. As I watched I gained a deeper connection to this whole family of beautiful birds and found forgiveness in my heart for Mr. Downer.

About the same time we had some wonderful cool days, unlike this week of scorching humidity. I was weary as usual from the doses of chemo running through my veins, zapping me of any energy or desire for activity. So there I sat on our front porch, reading and praying and listening, and observing the wonderful world at my doorstep. Birds of all kinds chirping and twittering as the wind was blowing—a wind that was cool, refreshing, and bending the green leafy branches of the aspens and lilacs. I felt good—close to God. And from my memory bank of special sayings from the Bible came these words:

> *The wind blows wherever it pleases. You hear its sound, but you cannot tell where it comes from or where it is going. So it is with everyone born of the Spirit.*
>
> ~John 3:8

That sure gave me lots to think about! Where I have come from and where I am going? These are quite tough issues to sort out, you know. Especially when you're sick! How did I get here and why? What could I have done to avoid being where I am? What more could I be doing now to move forward? And what does forward look like?

The key factor in the saying is the last statement: *"So it is with everyone born of the Spirit"*. Jesus put it this way in John 3, verse 7: "You must be born again". Even though I am longing for a new birth of health and energy, I realize that my real re-birth took place when I was only a seven year old. In a simple prayer of faith I asked Jesus Christ into my life. Since then, the winds of my life have blown in many directions, winds of change and winds of challenge. But it is the wind of the Spirit that has set the direction—and that has not and will not change.

Sometimes I have to admit to being confused. At the least I find it hard to reconcile certain oddities. On the one hand I am fully aware that I have personal responsibility to live my own life and make my own decisions. Life consists of actions and decisions for which only I can take ultimate responsibility. But on the other hand I am certain beyond the glimmer of a doubt that God is in control, ordering the events of my life and offering me *"everything I need for life and godliness"* (2 Peter 1:3). Let me share some of the context of that statement which has been an encouragement to me:

> *Grace and peace be yours in abundance through the knowledge of God and of Jesus our Lord. His divine power has given us everything we need for life and godliness through our knowledge of him who called us by his own glory and goodness. Through these he has given us his very great and precious promises.*

> ~2 Peter 1:2-4a

What more could we wish for?

TICKED OFF?

HAVE YOU EVER BEEN UPSET with God? Now come on! Be honest. I hope I'm not the only nerd on the planet. Surely you have had some reason at some time, going through some trying experience that has caused you not only to question God, but to get downright ticked off with Him. I know I'm not the only one, because recently I have been reading through the Psalms. David had his words with the Lord, and not only once— but many times. Remember that David was a warrior and being hunted down for extermination by his great enemy Saul. During those days he wrote many Psalms. He even accuses the Omnipresent One as being absent without leave—AWOL in army terms. Psalm 38:21 and the first verses of Psalm 10, 13, 22, 28, to mention a few.

Well, last week I had a day such as that. It was the first week of July, and I had my last "long" chemo treatment. Though happy to have it behind me, the reality of after effects was wearing me down in the midst of our heat wave. I did not write a Psalm, but I wrote a page in my diary and laid out some pretty clear complaints to the Lord.

I said (with a clearly angered and sarcastic tone in my pen): "Lord, how much more do I have to endure? Are you causing these awful chemicals to actually heal me? I feel like they are killing me! And what's on the agenda for my August 9 prostate check up? Lord, we are praying for healing and improvement with no further biopsy or treatments. Is that too much to ask? Or must you keep on accentuating my weakness to demonstrate your power? Lord, please have mercy on me."

At the bottom of each page of my journal is a printed verse of scripture. Almost overlooking it, my eye caught the reference in Zephaniah. "What in the world could a verse from that obscure part of the Bible, have to say to *me*," I thought. With a compassionate smile on His face and a firm arm around my shoulder, here is what God had to say to this frustrated, short-sighted follower.

> *The Lord your God is with you.*
> *He is mighty to save.*
> *He will take great delight in you.*
> *He will quiet you with His love.*
> *He will rejoice over you with singing.*
>
> ~Zephaniah 3:17

Now there is something to think about. Not only to think about, but to stuff into the memory bank for instant replay whenever things get out of perspective. I notice that there are no "ors" in the verse. It is not a list of things from which He chooses to bless me. I get the whole package. First, there are two great present tense truths about God—He is omnipresent and He is omnipotent (always with me and mighty to save). These are followed by three great promises. God delights in me, even though I can't see why He should. God quiets me with His love in the midst of uncertainty and frustration. And God sings to me, even though I'm temporarily a sidelined singer.

His songs have been wonderful. They are contained within the Psalms that I have been reading every day since that "down day". They go on and on and on telling me of His care and faithfulness. And I've noticed that David's complaints always led him to a stronger faith in God. So it is with me, and I trust for you as well.

I can't express how much everyone's prayers have meant to me. The last treatment is two weeks from tomorrow. Praise the Lord!

JUXTAPOSITION

NOW THERE'S AN INTERESTING WORD. It means "placed close together". It has an element of concurrence, or happening all at once, and with my limited vocabulary, I think of it as "layering".

It happened to me last night in the middle of a peaceful sleep. Awakened by the din of motorboats on Canal Lake which is a hundred or so meters from our back yard, I noticed it was past 2:00 a.m. What in the world were two or maybe three summer holiday fanatics doing barging rudely into my quiet space? The longer I lay there, the louder they seemed. My mind began to compose all sorts of questions. You know how it is in the middle of a sleepless night. How can they see out there to navigate? Are they part of the frightening statistics of drunk boaters? Don't they know people are TRYING TO SLEEP!

As a mild panic began to inject the hope that this roar of motors not be abruptly interrupted by an explosion or crash, I heard a whistle. Being a canoer of a sort, I understand the importance of carrying a whistle for emergency signaling. But this was no ordinary whistle. It was the crystal clear flute-like call of a loon, rising effortlessly in juxtaposition above the racket of the engines. The longer I listened, I realized this loon was relatively nearby and being answered by another, and yet another from farther away, and always lingering above the noise of the motors. My attention was fully diverted to these unique and beautiful water fowl that grace our environment.

Questions inundated my thoughts. This layering of midnight sounds in juxtaposition with each other got me thinking about my own life and present experience. My chemo therapy course is now finished. What a relief! What a joy to have known the enablement of the Lord and the encouragement of so many friends and family. But questions continued to escalate their noisy voices, motoring around the lake of my overactive imagination. Was the chemo effective? Will there need to be follow up of a similar sort? What other medical challenges lurk around the corner? When can I get back to work? Crowding one on the other with no clarity of resolution, I found these questions leading nowhere constructive.

Then like the piercing call of the loon, in juxtaposition to these disturbing messengers of doubt, came the voice of Jesus—not audibly, mind you, but out of my memory bank of verses learned in younger days.

Come to me, all of you who are weary and carry heavy burdens, and I will give you rest. Take my yoke upon you. Let me teach you, because I am humble and gentle, and you will find rest for your souls. For my yoke fits perfectly, and the burden I give you is light.

~Matthew 11:28-30 (NLT)

What a reminder of His grace! What a release from anxiety! Jesus, asking me to team up with Him, connect with Him, hook up to His wagon in tandem, side by side with the Prince of Peace, the Giver of Grace.

Caught up in these comforting thoughts, I heard the loon again far off in the distance. And the motor boats were gone. Everything was peaceful. Now each time the loon calls it becomes another reminder of Matthew 28—its voice in juxtaposition to that of my Saviour.

I hope those boaters finally had a peaceful sleep. My night was basically shot! But I ended up ready to take Jesus' prescribed rest which is bound to lead to better sleep.

GLORY MAKERS

HAVE YOU NOTICED HOW LIFE sometimes just plain loses its zest and glimmer? You must have heard of the dog days of summer. We had a few of them this summer with record breaking heat waves week after week. Frankly I've had enough of the hot stuff for this year, thank you very much!

Gardening has been a challenge for most people I'm sure, requiring regular watering and weeding during the cooler times of the day. As for me, I was told to avoid direct and intense sunlight during chemo therapy.

Last year was different. Cool days. Enjoying relatively good health. No struggle with lung cancer even though we were unaware it was lurking there, waiting for radical attention. And my garden! It thrived, especially the morning glories—big heavenly blue blossoms literally covering the trellis by our front door. Thousands of seeds fell into the fertile earth beneath, promising an even greater display for this year. Guess how many grew? Three! But that was exactly what I planted last year, so what's the problem?

This year they lost the glory! No flowers. Every day I go and check only to find green leaves wilting in the intense heat. They must feel like I have felt on many days. They certainly look like I look on far too many days. So what do you call a morning glory with no blossoms? Well, leaving out the glory and not finishing the word "blossoms" could leave us with "Morning Blahs". Or we could get downright nasty and call my morning un-glory plant "Ichabod"—meaning *"the glory has departed"*, taken from a dark chapter in the history of Israel. (1 Samuel 4:21)

Jesus had a similar experience with nothing but leaves. (Matthew 21:19) While out for a stroll with the disciples one day, he came upon a fig tree with no figs. Just leaves. What good is that? Jesus was not very impressed. Perhaps He saw the fig tree as a symbol of the people of God who were not producing the fruit of the Spirit—all caught up in a flurry of "useless leaves" but short on what really counts. This story really makes me think about myself. I am way too often like my gloryless morning glories, not displaying the beauty of the Lord as I am intended to do in my words and actions.

I have a host of glory makers to be thankful for. Caring health professionals have given me the best of care, looking after all the procedures and surgeries and chemo therapy of the past year. Now we're into follow-up assessment and observation. An army of friends and family have been encouraging me along the way with kind words and prayers. Our church family has been there for us throughout the whole ordeal. Sharon has been a wonderful wife and partner through it all, attending to my needs and even covering much of the music ministry in my absence.

We all need to be glory makers. Jesus wants us to let our light shine, to be morning glories for Him. Part of that mission is to focus on others and their needs, to do good things for people so that they too will "glorify" our Father in heaven. A smile. A kind word. A helpful hand. A friendly coffee. It all adds up to helping someone else become a glory maker. Sure is a lot better than being dubbed "Morning Blahs", and definitely way ahead of "Ichabod".

TIME TO THANK

LAST NIGHT I WAS THINKING back to our recent visit with Rob and Carina and our two grand-daughters. "Oh no, here he goes again", you say, "boring us with grandparent ravings". (That means "wild talk that makes no sense".) We'll see about that! In one week, and at only two weeks old, Kayleigh Anne had not only gained a part of a pound, but already her features had become more distinctly her. What a beautiful baby—a precious gift from our God. Then there's Amanda, who at 25 months old already *talks a blue streak*. We had given her a little baby doll which she immediately latched on to with moth-erly instinct. When I asked her how she liked her doll, she came close to me and gently said, "Thank you, Opa, for giving." Isn't that special!

One of the many weird sayings we have in English is "a blue streak". You've used it your-self, haven't you! To "talk a blue streak", means to "talk quickly and at an interminable length" about something. I retrieved this information on a chat line, and one person said that they were not certain of its exact etymology, but believe it somehow was related to a blue "streak of lightning" in the sense that someone who "talks a blue streak" is usually speaking on and on at a very fast rate. That would describe Amanda.

But isn't it special that her chosen words included thanksgiving. Don't you wish that we all would express thanks more spontaneously? Even to "thank a blue streak". Wouldn't that be something! Here we are on Thanksgiving Monday, many of us having listened yesterday to great sermons on being thankful in all things.

Always be thankful, for this is God's will for you who belong to Christ Jesus.

~1 Thessalonians 5:18 (NLT)

Frankly I don't know how that works or if I'm up to it. My mind reflected on the suffering in Pakistan, and Mexico, and New Orleans. We are surrounded by situations that cannot in any way be defined as good. But our Pastor reminded us that the "always" actually does include even the tough stuff of life, because God is intermingling all the circumstances of our lives into one big picture that ultimately brings glory to Him and good to us.

Even though I didn't overflow with gratitude every day (nor am I anywhere near such spiritual maturity), I have to thank God for bringing Sharon and me through this past year. Not what I would call the best year of my life, but a learning experience that has helped me put many things into perspective. One major part of my learning curve is to realize how many real friends are out there who, as representatives of Jesus himself, have taken time to pray, to write, to phone, to visit, to encourage, and to help.

Reports so far are good. I see my surgeon for follow-up next week, and am hopeful for more good news. My energy is returning. I volunteer some time each week preparing the choir for our series of five Christmas concerts. There is a torrent of things to be thankful for. Like David the Psalm writer said: *"I will praise my God to my last breath"*, (Psalm 104:33, NLT)—and so will I. I just don't want that day to come any sooner than God has planned it.

> *Give thanks to the Lord for He is good! His love endures forever. Who can list the glorious miracles of the Lord? Who can ever praise him half enough?*
>
> ~Psalm 106:1-2 (NLT)

Somehow we need to get a blue streak of thanksgiving going here. Maybe it's as simple as taking a lesson from Amanda.

MORNING AFTER SYNDROME

WELL, MY HEAD IS SPINNING TODAY!
You've heard of the morning after syndrome. I understand that it can be a real problem for folk who have over indulged the night before, apparently having had an exhilarating party, but needing a designated driver to get home, riding high on intoxication, only to wake up with a blazing headache and queasy stomach.

Well, last night I had a very exhilarating time—almost a party—and I did not need a designated driver to get me home. Nor did I wake up this morning with a blazing headache or queasy stomach. The only intoxication I had was exhilaration following the fifth of our series of Living Christmas Tree Concerts with attendance exceeding 3000. The finale said it all—"How Great Our Joy". Talk about up tempo! Calypso. Dancers. Flags flying. Lights flashing. Totally electrifying! As the audience applauded, we repeated the last half of the song with the audience joining in, singing and clapping, exploding with appreciation.

This final song summed up the theme of the concert, *Treasures of Christmas*. The dramatic portion depicted vandals who had stolen the baby Jesus doll. A street lady who had adopted the nativity scene as her place to sleep, carried on a hilarious but moving conversation with a shopper who was having a very bad day and hated Christmas. The street lady's classic comment was, *"It sounds like someone stole your Jesus too!"*

Jesus is the reason for the season. Jesus is the real treasure—the only truly valuable Christmas gift. By receiving Him, we end up with major bonuses: love, joy, and peace to mention only a few. But beyond that, we are given eternal life with absolute assurance that God has forgiven our sin and is preparing a place for us in heaven when this life comes to a close.

> *The free gift of God is eternal life, through Christ Jesus our Lord."*
>
> ~Romans 6:23 (NLT)

Yep! I was pumped. And today? Well my "morning after syndrome" is mixed with weariness and a sense of deep gratitude to God who has seen me through the most challenging of years. I am indebted to Him for giving me enough strength to carry out the leadership of this event. During the months of chemo therapy, I had spent time at home planning the concert. It gave me a sense of purpose and participation. How wonderful now, while still limited in time and energy, to have participated in this ministry during what would normally have been "time out".

January will be a month of more medical tests and updates. I know many of you reading this are going through the same thing. It isn't fun, is it? We always pray for good results. Naturally. Sometimes it is God's plan to heal us. Sometimes it isn't. But you know what? There's coming a morning when we will wake up realizing that the earthly party is over, and the "morning after syndrome" will be totally different. Streets of gold. Fresh air as never breathed before. Light and life, unending. Jesus, face to face. How great our joy will be!

TRULY POSITIVE AND EXHILARATING

WE'RE SO CONDITIONED to doom and gloom these days that we're taken by surprise when something truly positive and exhilarating occurs. The media digs deep to find "good news" stories, such as three men rescuing a baby moose from the ice, or someone discovering a cure for ingrown toenails! The best one I heard this week was that now they say coffee and chocolate are actually good for you. That may be stimulating for some of you, but I experienced something the other day that was truly positive and exhilarating. It gave me renewed courage and perspective.

You see, two days before that discovery (not the coffee and chocolate thing but the truly positive and exhilarating thing), I had been to the hospital to visit my surgeon. I asked him how he was and he said he was fine. Actually he's not the one we were worried about. It was me! Two weeks into 2006, here I am hoping to celebrate my one-year-after-lung-surgery anniversary. The question loomed as to whether we'd be singing "Happy Anniversary", or singing the blues.

After our initial greetings, it was a little intimidating to say the least as I waited to find out his latest prognosis. Digging deep in the rather voluminous file (like a news reporter looking for some uplifting news), he pulled out my CT Scan. "That's good", he said. Then out came the X-ray and up it went on the light screen. "That's good. No problem there." Then a little sheet marked Broncoscopy was retrieved. This was the test done just the day before, and the one I feared the most. I seized the moment and thanked him for putting me to sleep during the procedure as he had rammed the camera devise down my throat and into my bronchial tubes. For a moment my heart sank as I wondered if he was stalling for time. In a low voice he said, "I liked what I saw there yesterday". Thumping me on my back in several places, he assured me. "Sounds good. And you look good, too. Come and see me in four months".

Truly positive and exhilarating. But that's not what I started out to tell you. It was two days later when I made the awesome good news discovery. I was looking for a verse in the Bible to introduce a solo I was singing on Sunday: "My Father Watches Over Me". The song says it well, but the Bible says it better:

> Find rest, O my soul, in God alone.
> My hope comes from Him.
> He alone is my rock and my salvation.
> He is my fortress.

I will not be shaken.
My salvation and my honour depend on God.
He is my mighty rock, my refuge.
Trust in Him at all times, O people.
Pour out your hearts to Him, for God is our refuge.

~Psalm 62:5-8 (NIV)

Now isn't that something! Talk about good news. That's it. You can't beat having God as a resting place, a hiding place, and a safe place. And it wasn't written just for me. The last sentence opens the door for all of us. Truly positive and exhilarating!

UNDER SURVEILLANCE

WHEW! ALL IS WELL! No cancer in my prostate. "See me in six months. I want to keep you under surveillance!" That was the urologist's word for the day.

OK. OK. I'm a wimp! Wimps worry. And yesterday's consultation regarding my prostate biopsy had me pretty concerned. As I have mentioned before, I often experience a mixture of faith and fear when facing a doctor's report. Why is it we always seem to expect the worst and only vaguely hope for the best?

Sharon and I were commenting on how God is good no matter what. He is good, not only when we get these encouraging reports, but especially when we get bad news or have to go through tough times. When we are at our worst, God is at His best! The trick is learning to trust Him, always.

You see, I am not only under surveillance by my urologist, my thoracic surgeon, my oncologist, my respirologist, and my family doctor,—I am under God's surveillance. God is watching me. And not "from a distance" like the popular song says. He is very close. Very observant. Very interested in my circumstances. Why? Because in the same way he cares about you, he cares for me too.

So why do we worry so much? Why do I wimp out? I guess I need to be reminded again for the umpteenth time what the Master Wimp Buster said in Matthew Chapter 6:25-34:

> *Therefore I tell you, **do not worry** about your life, what you will eat or drink; or about your body, what you will wear (or its health!). Is not life more important than food, and the body more important than clothes (and perfect health)? Look at the birds of the air; they do not sow or reap or store away in barns, and yet your heavenly Father feeds them. Are you not much more valuable than they?*

> ***Who of you by worrying can add a single hour to his life?** (Good question!) And why do you worry about clothes? See how the lilies of the field grow. They do not labour or spin. Yet I tell you that not even Solomon in all his splendour was dressed like one of these. If that is how God clothes the grass of the field, which is here today and tomorrow is thrown into the fire, will he not much more clothe you, **O you of little faith?***

> ***So do not worry,** saying, 'What shall we eat?' or 'What shall we drink?' or 'What shall we wear?' (Or what if I get sick?) For the pagans (people who don't believe in God) run after all these things, and **your***

heavenly Father knows that you need them. But seek first his kingdom and his righteousness, and all these things will be given to you as well. **Therefore do not worry about tomorrow,** for tomorrow will worry about itself. Each day has enough trouble of its own.

SO, WHAT HAVE I LEARNED?

DURING 2005 I SENT OUT several short e-mail writings describing "My Journey of Hope" as I wandered through the experience of two lung surgeries and several months of chemotherapy. Then during the last couple of months it seems that my writings came to a screeching halt. Dried up. Probably recovery doldrums.

It is sometimes awkward when people ask how I am doing. "Fine" isn't always honest, but at least it's polite. In the back of my mind I'm thinking, "You don't really want to know". But more recently the most accurate response is, "Better". Some days, to be truthful, I would have to say, "Depressed". Others, I could honestly say, "Great". But let's be honest. I'm not the only one with ups and downs. I bet you're the same!

So what? Well, here's the scoop. The other day my pastor asked me a probing question. It was much more explicit than "How are you?". His question was: "What have you learned about yourself and about God?". I have to tell you that I hate those kinds of questions. I just don't think on my feet that fast. It's like those job interviews when they ask you what your greatest strength is. I usually say, "Duh"! To me, it is like trying to explain the universe!

My answers were really vague. I hardly remember what I said. (Maybe chemo has fried my memory bank!) But I do remember feeling very incompetent. I mean, if I haven't learned anything, then maybe I have failed in my Journey of Hope. No, I don't think so. But the question was a good one. Brilliant. And I hope I will figure out the answer—someday.

About the 'God' part, I remember saying that I didn't want to give a pat answer like "God is good all the time". I said that my view of God has not changed, and therefore I don't think I have learned anything about Him that I didn't know before. Even though that seems a bit arrogant, it's true. God has been my source of help and hope over many years. On a rather gentle learning curve I am figuring out how to trust God, often by hind sight more than foresight. You see, once you initially set out on a journey of following the Lord and trusting Him as leader of your life, it's on God's agenda to prove to you over and over that He can be trusted. Check it out. Wise old Solomon said it this way:

> *Trust in the LORD with all your heart and
> lean not on your own understanding;*
> *In all your ways acknowledge him, and he
> will make your paths straight.*

> ~Proverbs 3:5-6

The fact is that God permits us to suffer sometimes and uses that experience to confirm His loving kindness. I like *1 Peter 4:19*'s cut on it:

> *So then, those who suffer according to God's will should commit themselves to their faithful Creator and continue to do good.*

It is in the difficult times that we tend to pray more and turn to God more. That's a good thing. Even though He seemed closer to me in the darkest hours, in reality He is always near. So there's a thumbnail sketch of my faith walk. I'm sure God has lots more to teach me about Himself.

But what have I learned about myself? "Duh". I'm too much the same as I was before. Flawed. But that's OK because God loves flawed people. He died for flawed people. Romans 5:8 says:

> *God demonstrated His own love for us in this: While we were still sinners, Christ died for us.*

And more than that—He has prepared a way for flawed people to go to heaven. It is there that we will find out that our learning has only just begun.

So yeah, I'm doing fine.

WELL-BEING ISN'T ALWAYS BEING WELL!

DURING THE LAST THREE MONTHS I have had yet another round of checkups, x-rays, CT scan, and blood tests followed by consultations by Dr. K., Dr. A., Dr. B., Dr. T. and Dr. S. The next round begins in August. Praise God that all reports so far have been encouraging. I was going to say 'excellent' but my inner voice is arguing, *not permitting my being well to be defined as well-being.* Isn't it crazy how we can't accept good things face value? I know I have a problem there. Instead, I find myself doubting and dredging up the proverbial "what ifs", and dwelling on minutiae. Maybe I'm unique in all that. Probably not. I hope not.

I seem to be in some sort of slump, even though I have had excellent reports from my doctors. My inner dialogue goes something like this: "So what—if Dr. B. oncologist used words like, 'fabulous, incredible, and remarkable"? Why then would both he and Dr. K. recommend that I not be in a hurry to return to full time work? And so what—if Dr. S. urologist is pleased that my PSA dropped, even if it was less than one point? Why do I have to get checked again in 3 months? And what will Dr. A. respirologist say next week, and Dr. T. surgeon the next?

My heart says I want to go back to work again, but my head and body don't fully agree. Others have also told me not to be in a hurry. It looks like I will continue volunteering at the church for around 15 hours a week.

During the past year I have communicated much in my letters regarding my Journey of Hope. The ups and downs. The laughter and pain. The tough days and the good days. And today, instead of jumping for joy, I seem to be caught like a ship in the doldrums (defined as a period of stagnation or slump, or a period of depression or unhappy listlessness).

There is an equatorial area of calm know as the doldrums located slightly north of the equator, and spanning the earth between the two belts of trade winds. The doldrums are noted for periods when the winds disappear, trapping sailing vessels for days or weeks. Early sailors named this belt of calm the "doldrums" because of the low spirits they found themselves in after days of no wind.

This is definitely not like the apostle Paul who said in Philippians 4:12-13:

I have learned the secret of being content in any and every situation, whether well fed or hungry, whether living in plenty or in want. I can do everything through him who gives me strength.

I desperately need God's strength and the wind of his Spirit in my sails.

The other day I was reading in *Romans 12*, and when I arrived at verse 12 the Lord gave me a very practical self-help assignment. He said:

> *Be joyful in hope, patient in affliction, faithful in prayer.*

Now that gives me something worthwhile to get my head and my heart around, and to translate into action..

So I guess *well-being isn't always a matter of being well*. I thank God for my health. But I have so much yet to learn. I love the Lord, and I know he loves me. I am not doubting Him, not even for a moment. I am only getting impatient with schedules and circumstances. My hope is that God will be patient with me because they say those doldrums are also spawning grounds for hurricanes, and I've had enough storms—at least for now!

FISHCAPADE

I LOVE THOSE STORIES in the Bible about fishing (see below). Peter, James and John were *real* fishermen. They knew how and when and where, and probably had their reason why. But today I can't imagine why anyone would want to waste time trying to snag those slippery, slimy critters.

Today was my first fishing escapade since returning from Prince George, BC in 2000. Out there fishing was such great fun. We almost always came back with our full quota of rainbow trout. Tasty! And plenty to freeze for later as well. I had acquired a small aluminum boat which I named "Catch 22", that was modestly equipped with a small electric fishing motor and a set of oars just in case the battery failed. My fishing gear is more modest than my boat was. I say 'was' because the boat and motor were among the myriad of things we left behind when we moved here. But my pitiful fishing gear was carefully packed and never used until today.

Today, six years later, I decided that it was high time to go fishing again. I finally invested in a fishing license about a month ago anticipating this momentous day. I thought it would be good therapy for me since there are many days that need to be filled with meaningful, energizing and up-building activities. By the way, my latest round of medical reports proved to be very encouraging, and no more are scheduled until mid October.

So what better way to spend a day than on the lake. Canal Lake is only about 150 yards from our house. I have a canoe that we portage to the lake. Prior to my surgeries I had no difficulty lifting it up on my shoulders and carrying it. I had tested this procedure a few weeks ago and was confident that I could get there by myself.

First, I had to get my gear ready. What a mess! Tangled fish line has to be the worst frustration life can dish out. Then I needed some rope for which I searched endlessly and unsuccessfully, only to be found by phoning Sharon at work asking for her help. That being solved, I proceeded to put a small lunch together, get my sun glasses, life jacket, paddle, and a canvass bag to rig up some sort of anchor. Rocks in a bag seemed to make sense. Realize that I have never fished from a canoe before. All this I carried to the shore of the lake and returned to the house for my canoe. With a sense of pride and well-being I lifted the canoe to my shoulders and portaged to the lake, trying not to look too rickety in case someone was watching.

As I made my way across the grassy access to the lake, my mind drifted to our younger son

Marty and his wife Holly who are entertainers on a cruise ship somewhere off the shores of Alaska. They don't have to carry their boat! It carries them. They don't have to fish for meals. Theirs are prepared and served by the crew. What a life! What an adventure! However, not near the adventure I was about to experience. My day dream suddenly ended and I was at the shore.

I loaded everything into the canoe, tying the rope in an intricate way with one end tethering the anchor and the other tied to my tackle box and both tied to the canoe, just in case the canoe happened to capsize. I didn't want to lose anything—especially my pitiful fishing gear. The exciting moment of launch came and went, only to reveal that I had launched it backwards. I'm used to canoeing with a partner and seldom go alone. Solo canoeing requires turning the canoe around and using what is usually the front seat as the back seat. Shoving it back on to the bank, I then had to untie and re-tie everything on the opposite, proper end.

That finally done, I got in and paddled serenely out into the lake a short distance and let down my make-shift rocks-in-a-bag anchor. It worked perfectly. Then worming my hook I cast out into the deep and caught nothing—just like Jesus' disciples. I didn't even have to be told to try casting on the other side. I tried the left, the right, the front and the back—several times! Nothing. Only lots of sea weed on my lure. Oh, I had a few bites. They ate about three of my worms. Then bang! I got one! It tugged and tugged relentlessly until I landed it in the boat— a sunfish about four inches long. And that was it. Not much of a meal there!

But just then four recreational boats came storming by. I realized that their wake was going to be pretty big so I tried to steer the canoe toward them, but the anchor was holding me. So scrambling with all my might I quickly pulled up the bag of rocks just in time and got the canoe turned to face the waves. Whew!

Then I decided to fish without the anchor and drift. There was a bigger breeze than I realized and in no time I was halfway across the lake! Paddling like the blazes I tried desperately to turn around, but the wind was bent on driving the front end of the canoe east instead of west. Well, I persisted and finally got turned, heading straight for home (against the wind, of course). It was a great challenge.

To my dismay, someone was watching me. Yes, I know Jesus was,—thankfully! But so was someone else. Our neighbour was standing there observing my awkward canoeing technique and probably wondering who in the world would go fishing in a canoe on a windy day on a lake occupied by big pleasure boats with huge wakes, all by himself. That would be me, of course!

So what is the moral of this story? I don't know! You figure it out! I guess for me I am left with three questions: What ever possessed me to buy a fishing license in the first place? What better way to spend a day than golfing? Yes, I said golfing. Forget fishing! And third, why do those poor little worms have to suffer so much for so little? Well, my canoe is back where it belongs—under the deck. I think I'll name it "Catch the wind".

———   ———   ———

Here's one of those stories I love so much. I relate somewhat to Peter. Notice Jesus' compassion in reassigning Peter to a new job—not fishing! His boat resting dry as a sand dollar on the shore says it all.

> One day as Jesus was standing by the Lake of Gennesaret, with the people crowding around him and listening to the word of God, he saw at the water's edge two boats, left there by the fishermen, who were washing their nets. He got into one of the boats, the one belonging to Simon, and asked him to put out a little from shore. Then he sat down and taught the people from the boat.
>
> When he had finished speaking, he said to Simon, "Put out into deep water, and let down the nets for a catch." Simon answered, "Master, we've worked hard all night and haven't caught anything. But because you say so, I will let down the nets." When they had done so, they caught such a large number of fish that their nets began to break.

So they signaled their partners in the other boat to come and help them, and they came and filled both boats so full that they began to sink. When Simon Peter saw this, he fell at Jesus' knees and said, "Go away from me, Lord; I am a sinful man!" For he and all his companions were astonished at the catch of fish they had taken, and so were James and John, the sons of Zebedee, Simon's partners. Then Jesus said to Simon, "Don't be afraid; from now on you will catch men." So they pulled their boats up on shore, left everything and followed him.

~Luke 5:1-11

BLUE BONNET DEPRESSION

I DON'T THINK I EVER told you about the skunk! One day we saw this funny looking skunk with a blue head wandering aimlessly around our driveway and yard. Not wanting to get close to it for obvious reasons, I got out my binoculars because this was the funniest skunk I had ever seen. Upon closer yet distant observation, I was horrified to see that it had a plastic "Blue Bonnet" margarine container stuck on its face. The skunk pushed the container into the ground everywhere it went, obviously not having a clue where it was going. I could just sense that this was one very depressed and frustrated old skunk!

Brave as I am, I set out at once to figure out a way to fix this problem. So mustering up courage I opened the door, but then with great determination decided to call the humane society instead! They told me it would cost $75 for them to come, but they couldn't be sure they would even find it when they got here. We were leaving to go to a birthday party, so I resorted to prayer. I prayed for a skunk! Well, I couldn't get close enough to counsel it, so prayer is all I had to give. We never saw the skunk again, unless it is the same one (minus the margarine container) that has been rooting up my yard.

Some days I feel like that very depressed and frustrated old skunk. Life just stinks! And I can't see where I am going. Even though more than a year has passed since the end of my chemo treatments, I feel energy deprived. Another health challenged person reminded me the other day that we will never be the same as we were. So true. Life goes on and things happen, change challenges us, and physically we're just not the same. We try to be. At least I have tried to be. But those expectations are nasty task masters. I sometimes get depressed when I reach my limit before I have reached my goal.

That was the case last week,—yet another one of those yucky weeks. I thought by now that I would be up and running like the Duracell Bunny, or at least like a skunk with no container on his head. But things are *not* the same. Life *has* changed a great deal in the past two years. Goals I had set in place should have been accomplished by now, but they're not. Even if I had the opportunity to re-address them, I have neither the capacity nor the inner motivation to achieve them. Do you know what I mean? Maybe you have been there. Maybe you are with me in this right now.

I can't imagine what deep depression is like. I have recently experienced mild to medium depression and it isn't fun! Every morning after a lousy sleep, waking up only to descend into a black hole of despair and sadness is the pits. All the while I blame myself, my spiritual immaturity, my laziness, my inability to cope with the slightest annoyance. It gets murkier the more the personal excuses over-ride the physical realities.

But yeah, everybody tells me I'm looking well. They say, "How are you doing? You're looking great". And I just respond, "Pretty good". And that's true. And pretty good is OK. Matter of fact, compared to large segments of the world's population, 'pretty good' is really good. So thank the Lord for 'pretty good'. But good on the outside is often not good on the inside. So how do we deal with this depression thing? How do we get the Blue Bonnet off our face?

Well, I pray a lot. These aren't 'on my knees' prayers. Maybe they should be, but I tend to converse with the Lord throughout the day, asking for help, for relief, for healing and mercy and grace and all the good things He has for us. God continues to use the Book of Philippians, which I know by memory, to prod me about so many things. For example:

> *Do not be anxious about anything, but in everything, by prayer and petition, with thanksgiving, present your requests to God. And the peace of God, which transcends all understanding, will guard your hearts and your minds in Christ Jesus.*
>
> ~Philippians 4:6-7

Looking back, I see where He *has* delivered the goods so graciously, just at the right time in the right way, to bring me through. But He hasn't protected me from the hurt and discomfort of the process. I think it is on the anvil of process that we are shaped. And the shaping process really hurts sometimes.

On "Who Wants To Be A Millionaire" one of the lifelines is 'Phone a Friend'. God has helped me through my own 'Phone a Friend' lifeline. The counsel and encouragement of friends are great benefits—worth much more than a million dollars. The best counsellors are often trusted friends and their advice is like sweet perfume. That has been the case for me. Proverbs 27:9 says:

> *Perfume and incense bring joy to the heart,*
> *and the pleasantness of one's friend springs*
> *from his earnest counsel.*

One of my trusted friends recently invested a lot of his valuable time in helping me gain some perspective. That very night I slept well. Pains that had racked my body diminished. I woke up refreshed and the black hole turned to grey. I think I know where I am going now. I realize that things are never going to be the same as they were. That's life. That's what I have to embrace. Thank God I don't have to call the Humane Society to take off my Blue Bonnet.

VISUALLY IMPAIRED

SOME FOLK HAVE SAID that November was typically dull and gray. Not for me. Maybe it was a bit gray. Certainly it wasn't dull, because we have been preparing for our Living Christmas Tree Concerts in mid December. Five concerts on one weekend. Yikes! And that's two weeks from now.

The other un-dull thing was getting a really good word from Dr. T. surgeon. Looking intently into my recent CT scan and comparing it to a year ago, he said: "Well I don't see any cancer growing in there. Looks good!" Praise to God exploded deep in my heart. Hindsight helps us compare where we are with where we were a year or two ago, gaining perspective and seeing what changes may or may not be taking place in our lives. Honest perspective then helps in our foresight, but it requires eyes that are willing to see.

Speaking of eyesight, years ago I had a singing student who was blind. I guess, for some unclear reason, we are to say "visually impaired". He was really fun to be with. Always joking about something. I would listen patiently to his lengthy tales, which ate up valuable lesson time, responding verbally to him rather than nodding my unseen head. I would interject, "I see". He would say: "I know you see. You're lucky". Then I would say, "But you see, we need to get back to the lesson". And he would say, "No I don't see", and then laugh.

You see (there I go again!) when we say "we see", it can mean so many things. It can mean we understand, or we visually behold it. It can mean we notice something, or simply that we "get it".

Well, this week I gained a new appreciation of what sight is all about. During recent months, I have been having problems seeing clearly. It wasn't just that gray November either. Occasionally the choir was wondering if I was losing it (not my eyesight!), when I would say we are on page 53 and it was actually 88. It appeared I was either confused, careless, suffering from chemo-brain, or impaired. But all you seniors know what I mean—visually challenged.

Last week the optometrist found cataracts behind my eyes that need to be removed some-time in the new year. That's OK. I'm used to medical procedures. Even though they seem to be taking me away gradually by bits and pieces, I don't feel diminished at all. I'm just thrilled they can do these things. I don't see print and signs clearly right now. But neither do I see the big picture of life. It's like having spiritual cata-racts which hamper my vision of what God is doing in this world and particularly in my life. I was pondering I Corinthians 13:12:

> *Now we see but a poor reflection as in a mirror; then we shall see face to face.*

The Greek word "ainigma" in this sentence means "an obscure saying, or enigma". There are many things I don't understand about the Bible and Jesus. Some things we won't understand until we get to heaven. But I love the fact that some day in the future—maybe not too distant—the cataracts of this gray world view will drop like scales and we will see Him face to face.

Spiritual blindness is a totally bigger malady. Jesus said:

> *"Do you have eyes but fail to see, and ears but fail to hear? And don't you remember?"*
>
> ~Mark 8:18

It was a direct hit on his followers who had already forgotten his miraculous power to feed great crowds of people with next to no food on hand. They were too blind to see who was right in front of them—the Messiah, who that same day would open both the physical and spiritual eyes of a blind man. Spiritual blindness obscures God from the picture entirely, and nobody wants to face life that way. Allowing God to open our eyes, we can see Jesus and His love and forgiveness.

Did you ever notice in the Bible how often Jesus commands us to *"Behold"* or *"Watch"*?

Good reminders to be vigilant and alert to what's really important. Keep your eyes open!

VACATION THERAPY

AREN'T VACATIONS WONDERFUL? I'm convinced they're a God thing. Even Jesus invited his followers to get away:

> *"Come with me by yourselves to a quiet place and get some rest." So they went away by themselves in a boat to a solitary place.*
>
> ~Mark 6:31-32

We just got back from a week in South Carolina. It was an . . . interesting week. A good time, but a bit cold most days. Walking on the beach wearing my fleecy "Canada" coat felt a little silly until we saw a lady with a heavy ankle-length wool coat buttoned up to her chin. By the end of the week we enjoyed some nice warm and sunny days. But I have to tell you about what made the experience "interesting".

You see, I don't see all that well. These cataracts that I mentioned in my last letter are not improving. They're not expected to until they are gone. Having an extra driver was not the only reason we brought Brian and Sharon Seeley along with us. They are good friends from HCJB with whom we served in Ecuador back in the mid 70's and early 80's. True, my Sharon was concerned that I have help with the driving. The eye surgeon had told me my bad eye was already under the legal limit for driving. One thousand miles is a long way for a half blind driver!

Well, I took the driver's seat for the first leg of the journey which included the border. Borders are really intimidating—even when you are innocent. I had nervously rehearsed what I should say and what I should refrain from saying, when suddenly we were ready to move forward to the inspector. But in my panic, I couldn't for the life of me figure out how to put the window down. You see, we had rented a larger car—a Buick Alure. Nice car, but I hadn't rehearsed how to work all the buttons.

In the nick of time I found out that by pushing on a little gizmo, my window came down. And there staring through that blessed empty space was the officer, ready to interrogate me. After scrutinizing our documents, he told us to have a nice day.

Nice Day? It was raining buckets! But that's not all. In a multi-tasked manner squinting at the highway signs, replacing my documents, poking at this and that trying to get the window back up, I accidentally put all the windows down! The rain came blowing in from all sides as Brian and Sharon and my Sharon burst into reams of laughter. Vehicles seemed to be coming from every direction and the main highway loomed in front of me. I'm pushing and pulling everything I can find. Finally I made for the side of the highway and figured the crazy thing out. Easy. Push down for down. Lift up for up. I'm not only visually challenged—I'm obviously challenged in other ways as well.

Brian took over after awhile. It was quite foggy and dismal. No breath taking scenery to speak of. God's creation takes on a misty, blurry look when it's raining—similar to how things look through cataracts. So I commented to the others how pleased I was, because now I wasn't the only one to miss out on the nice scenery! I guess that wasn't a nice thing to say. Anyway, while Brian drove, this was my chance to check out all the interesting switches and buttons. I couldn't see what was written on them so it was a trial and error kind of experimentation that went on for many miles. Sometimes spoken aloud, sometimes to myself: "I wonder what happens if I push this—or that?"

Along the way Brian commented that there was something wrong with the speedometer. (Try telling that to a policeman!) He had been going along about 110 km/hr figuring that was around 65 mph. But now it was registering down around 55 or 60. He sped up a bit and began to pass the traffic. It was obvious that 80 felt a little rushed and there was no way he was going to get it back up to 110 without becoming airborne. Deciding the speedometer was broken, we drove on—now with the extra worry of having a repair bill to pay when we get back. A little farther down the road, we realized that in my experimentation I had switched the odometer from kilometers to miles. What a great invention. Nice to be emerging from the dark ages!

I don't have time nor space nor desire to go into further detail about what made the week interesting, except to say that getting away was good therapy. It's a God thing. Why not do it where there is a sandy beach handy?

ON THE SHELF?

SOMETHING ISN'T QUITE RIGHT. It's June and my canoe is still in its perch in the garage, and my golf clubs are hiding under the steps.

I can understand the canoe being reluctant to get down off the shelf after treating me so badly last summer during my one and only fishing escapade. Who would have thought that any canoe in its right mind would allow anyone to try fishing while bobbing and turning, and being driven by unrelenting winds and bombarded with giant wakes from passing pleasure craft? My poor, lonely canoe is probably quite relieved to "stay put".

The golf clubs are a different matter. They represent relaxation and contentment, things that have been in rather short supply during recent weeks and months. Someday soon I am going to drop everything and get them both into action again. Not at the same time, mind you!

So what has been occupying our time and attention? Medical appointments. Church ministry. Family functions. All critically important. But overlapping everything, a huge decision to consider retirement.

After I had publicly announced my resignation one Sunday morning, someone asked me how I felt. I said I felt rather sad. We will be leaving many great friends and a meaningful music ministry behind. Truth is, I'm much like the canoe and golf clubs. On the shelf. Packed away for future use.

Not to worry! Life will go on, the greens will be greener, and the fish might even start biting. Many folk have reminded us that the Lord has a wonderful plan for our lives. It comes across a bit cliché-ish, but it is true nonetheless. I have walked a life of faith long enough to realize that God really cares for you and me. He knows the future and wants to walk with us into it. When I was a kid, we used to sing a song that says: *"My Lord knows the way through the wilderness. All I have to do is follow"*. You might rightfully ask, "What does that look like! How do we put wheels on it?" Wise old Solomon put it this way:

In all your ways acknowledge Him and He will make your paths straight.

~Proverbs 3:6

In other words, acknowledge God's desire to help us in our point of need. Acknowledge Jesus as He promises salvation, a gift simply to be accepted. Acknowledge our own scarcity compared to His incredible adequacy.

So what's next? First we must sell our house. Then we plan to move back to the city where

Sharon and I met and went to college together. How romantic is that!! London. (Ontario, that is.) It is central to all our siblings, and not far from our son Rob and his wife, Carina, and our two lovely granddaughters, Amanda and Kayleigh. We would also like to be closer to our other son Marty and his wife, Holly, but they are located wherever in the world the cruise ship, on which they work, takes them!

Remember my cataracts which I wrote about last December? One got fixed in March and the other one is scheduled for June 26. It will be nice to be less visually impaired. As for my lung cancer, the surgeon has now moved me to annual instead of three month surveillance. I expect the oncologist, who I see day after tomorrow, will be transferring my files to another oncologist in London since there are several things that need to be watched closely. I am so grateful for improved health and for the prayers and expressions of support from so many people. I have felt the closeness of God through it all.

Someday soon I may just wrestle that canoe off its perch and portage it to the lake. That's good exercise for the lungs! And before we move away from here, I'd better dust off those golf clubs and pay at least one more visit to the Greens. Perhaps in so doing, it will help me get down off the shelf, too.

SQUINTING'S OVER

EVEN AFTER TWO OR THREE YEARS of blurry vision due to the onset of cataracts, I'm still not sure whether squinting actually works. I've had lots of practice, much to the chagrin of my dear wife Sharon. Whenever I would try to see things more clearly, I was either nudged quietly when in public or told firmly if in private, "Stop squinting". It bothered her that I looked so weird with a pained expression on my face all wrinkled up and my eyes half shut. That's the funny part. Why do we shut our eyes when we try to see things more clearly? It makes no sense.

The other day I went for a long walk. The air was cool. Everything was particularly and unusually beautiful. The sun was bright. Very bright, and I realized that I wasn't squinting. My second new lens had been inserted on June 26. Now I enjoy Cataracts replaced by Cadillacs—the best on the market, worth every penny of the $535 each (not covered by OHIP). Hurray, I can see again. I began to notice the wild daisies, not just the flowers but the little white petals gleaming in the sunshine. The sky was the bluest ever—brilliant, almost incandescent, with contrasting cumulus clouds (dark on the bottom and billowing white cotton on top). Wow! Does everybody see all this in this same hew and texture?

That's when I started reminiscing about my squinting habit. Sharon was convinced it was a habit. Squinting is so nonsensical. Everybody does it when you go to the optometrist and they make you tell them what the little letters are. After Eye #1 cataract was done, still hampered by old Eye #2, I had squinted my way down to the 2nd or 3rd line from the bottom of the chart. "How did I do?", I asked the doctor. "You had eight wrong", he retorted blandly. The other day with both my eyes fixed, the surgeon said, "Good. You will be able to drive without glasses now. That is, if you have a license". Woops! I had been already doing that for the last two months, that is driving without glasses and squinting, and with a license.

I had a friend share with me via e-mail a word of encouragement. He said: "I make one prayer for you at any time I bring my concern for you before the Holy Spirit: that you will know God's purpose in it all. Everything falls into place when we have that assurance. That is, after all, how we regard even death." Thanks Morrison!

God is far sighted. He sees the end from the beginning. I am near sighted. The future is blurry. Squinting doesn't help at all. Matter of fact, I'd better keep both eyes wide open.

Whether we are near sighted or far sighted, it is a good thing to be able to decipher things clearly. I have often been too near sighted to see the big picture. Even though I know God has a purpose in our going through cancer and stuff, I have often found it too easy to focus on myself and not on God. I don't want to be like those folk Jeremiah wrote about,

> *"Hear this, you foolish and senseless people,*
> *who have eyes but do not see. . ."*
>
> ~Jeremiah 5:21

I want my spiritual eyes to see clearly—just as clearly as my new lenses. I want to see myself clearly. All the flaws that need worked on. All my potential that needs mobilized. All my capacity to care for and help others. To see God's purpose, and decipher my role in it.

A song we used to sing during our ministry in Ecuador was: "Let me see this world, dear Lord, as though I were looking through your eyes". Now, that's a challenge. For sure it's not for squinters. Let's keep both eyes open—and smile!

TOONIE LOONS

WAKING UP REFRESHED IS WONDERFUL. Doesn't happen every day, but July 10 was one of those mornings. My first awareness was a loon way out in the middle of Canal Lake conversing with a mourning dove on a nearby branch outside our bedroom window. L-looon- looon-looon. Hoo-dloooo-coo-coo-coo. A squawking crow joined in—Caw-caw-caw, followed by what seemed to be a myriad of fanciful fowl chirping and twittering their little hearts out. Too often I doze through that incredible symphony of the rising sun.

We're going to miss our home in Bolsover. Situated only a hundred meters from Canal Lake, and surrounded on three sides by woodland, our house is nestled snugly in the habitat of some of God's neatest little creatures. Skunks, squirrels, chipmunks, porcupines, and birds galore,—woodpeckers, wrens, red and yellow finches, sparrows, robins, Baltimore orioles, to name only a few. A rose breasted grosbeak has been entertaining me at the birdfeeder this week. Within a few kilometers is the protected Carden

Bird Sanctuary, little-known and not recognized by the general public. But the loons always capture my admiration. No wonder they grace our "loonie".

I've learned a lot, these last seven years from our wooded vantage point. God has used his creation both to cheer me and to teach me about myself, especially during my health struggles. Mr. Downer, the downy woodpecker with his incessant rat-a-tat-tating on my eaves trough during my fight with cancer and chemo therapy, taught me that he could be even more annoying than my worst chemo day. The ugly, unmannered grackles scaring away those innocent little finches, showed me how not to nurture relationships. Poor Mrs. Blue Bonnet, the skunk with a margarine container stuck over her face (the funniest tragic thing I ever saw), caused me to take a closer look at depression. She was in far worse shape than I.

Last week was the best ever. A viewing of our 'house for sale' required me to be gone for an hour, so I went fishing. I was having so much fun that it ended up being three hours. No, I didn't take the canoe this time! I stood safely on the shore. But listen to what happened. All of a sudden I heard this flapping, flailing, fluttering sound coming towards me. Looking up, I saw two loons, side by side, suspended between heaven and earth, appearing to be trying to take off into flight, but dragging their feet in the water. They were covering several hundred yards very quickly, neither air borne nor water logged, with their wing tips thrashing the water as they flew. Then as quickly as they appeared, those two loonies were out of sight. It was really strange. I pondered the weirdness of it while reeling in my tiny catch of the day that was hardly worth gutting, scaling and cooking. But guess what happened! The people who were looking at our house, bought it!

Now, what in the world does that have to do with anything? I'm not sure. But all of a sudden our life has started to take off. No more sitting in our secluded, almost predictable haven. We have seen so many answers to long standing prayers during the past week or so! My cataracts are done and gone. Our house sold. Our new house in London purchased. Moving date is August 17—exactly as we had hoped and prayed. It seems everything is happening all at once.

Here we are, wings flapping in forward motion like those two loons suspended between heaven and earth. Our feet are wet in the reality of life-changing decisions. Our focus is upward as we trust God for the unknowns of our future. Trusting God sometimes means waiting a long time for answers to prayers. Sometimes it means making the effort to move forward even when our feet seem to be dragging in the water. Remember the story in Matthew's Gospel when Peter walked on the water with Jesus? He discovered that taking his eyes off the Lord got him very wet.

> *Jumping out of the boat, Peter walked on the water to Jesus. But when he looked down at the waves churning beneath his feet, he lost his nerve and started to sink. He cried, "Master, save me!"*
>
> ~Matthew 14:22-33

Truth is, you and I both can depend on God helping us, especially when we ask Him to.

> *Look at the birds of the air; they do not sow or reap or store away in barns, and yet your heavenly Father feeds them. Are you not much more valuable than they?*
>
> ~Jesus, Matthew 6:26

Good question! I like those loons and they seem pretty valuable to me.

EPILOGUE

LIFE GOES ON. And guess what? Odds are we'll be visited by more sickness, and we'll be visiting more doctors perhaps sooner than we think. It is all part of being human. I can personally admit to being blessed by sickness. "Blessed?", you say. Yes, blessed. Through it my world has expanded rather than contracted. I now have firsthand experience with our great Canadian medical system. And I have no complaints. I have a greater empathy and understanding of what so many go through who are much sicker than I ever was. I have more friends and better friends who share at a deeper level. I have drawn closer to God than ever before. Even the valley experiences have given deeper joy and a greater appreciation for life than we get from the mountaintop highs often associated with health, wealth and happiness.

Our move to London is a major turning point in our lives. A new chapter begins. New surroundings. New friends. New doctors! I expect it will take some getting used to. I also expect the magazines in the medical clinic waiting rooms will be more or less the same!

But one thing is for certain. No matter how many years or decades I live in London, there is a better home waiting beyond the horizon. God has prepared a place for all who see beyond the immediate and look towards heaven through eyes of faith in Jesus. It is so easy to get distracted from the main thing, to be caught up in whatever challenges life dishes out, forgetting that this world is not our ultimate home.

> *But our citizenship is in heaven. And we eagerly await a Savior from there, the Lord Jesus Christ, who, by the power that enables Him to bring everything under His control, will transform our lowly bodies so that they will be like His glorious body.*
>
> ~Philippians 3:20-21

Printed in the United States
101917LV00001B/16-96/P

9 781897 373187